EMPOWERED STRATEGIES

FOR

MAXIMIZING

HEALTH

Exploring the Benefits of Ample Vitamin D, Vitamin C, and Iodine.

Taylor Francis

DISCLAIMER

TABLE OF CONTENTS

INTRODUCTION

Nutrients are the substances that our body needs to function properly and stay healthy. They include vitamins, minerals, amino acids, fatty acids, and other compounds that are essential for various biological processes. However, nutrients do not work in isolation. They interact with each other in complex and dynamic ways, influencing their availability, absorption, and utilization in the body. This phenomenon is known as nutrient synergy. Nutrient synergy is the concept that the combined effects of two or more nutrients are greater than the sum of their individual effects. In other words, nutrients can enhance or inhibit each other's actions, depending on the context and the dose. For example, vitamin C can increase the absorption of iron from plant sources, while calcium can reduce it. Similarly, vitamin D can enhance the absorption of calcium and phosphorus, while magnesium can regulate their metabolism. Understanding nutrient synergy is important for optimizing our health and well-being. By knowing how nutrients interact with each other, we can make better dietary choices and supplement decisions that suit our individual needs and goals. Moreover, nutrient synergy can help us prevent or treat various diseases and conditions that are caused or influenced by nutrient imbalances or deficiencies. For instance, vitamin D, vitamin C, and iodine are three nutrients that play vital roles in our immune system, bone health, and thyroid function, respectively. By ensuring adequate intake and synergy of these nutrients, we can boost our immunity, prevent osteoporosis, and support our metabolism.

In this book, we will explore the benefits of ample vitamin D, vitamin C, and iodine for our health and wellness. We will also unveil the sources, factors, and strategies that affect their availability, absorption, and utilization in our body. Finally, we will provide practical tips and recommendations on how to craft a balanced diet that integrates these nutrients in optimal amounts and ratios. By the end of this book, you will have a deeper understanding of nutrient synergy and how to harness its power for your health journey.

The Interplay of Vitamins and Minerals

Vitamins and minerals are two types of nutrients that are essential for our health. Vitamins are organic substances that the body needs in trace amounts for a variety of metabolic processes. Minerals are inorganic elements that are involved in various physiological functions, such as nerve transmission, muscle contraction, and fluid balance. There are 13 vitamins and 16 minerals that are recognized as essential for human health. Vitamins and minerals can be classified into two groups based on their solubility: water-soluble and fat-soluble. Water-soluble vitamins include vitamin C and the B-complex vitamins, such as thiamine, riboflavin, niacin, pantothenic acid, biotin, folate, and cobalamin. These vitamins are dissolved in water and are easily absorbed and excreted by the body. They need to be consumed regularly, as they are not stored in significant amounts in the body. Fat-soluble vitamins include vitamins A, D, E, and K. These vitamins are dissolved in fat and are absorbed with the help of bile and lipases. They are stored in the liver and adipose tissue and can accumulate to toxic levels if consumed in excess.

Vitamins and minerals interact with each other in complex and dynamic ways, influencing their availability, absorption, and utilization in the body. Some of these interactions are synergistic, meaning that they enhance each other's effects. For example, vitamin C can increase the absorption of iron from plant sources, while vitamin D can enhance the absorption of calcium and phosphorus. Some of these interactions are antagonistic, meaning that they inhibit each other's effects. For example, calcium can reduce the absorption of iron, zinc, and magnesium, while vitamin A can interfere with the metabolism of vitamin K.

The interplay of vitamins and minerals is influenced by various factors, such as the source, form, dose, timing, and combination of the nutrients, as well as the individual's age, gender, health status, and genetic variations. Therefore, it is important to consider the whole picture of nutrient synergy when planning a balanced and varied diet that meets the recommended dietary allowances (RDAs) and tolerable upper intake levels (ULs) of each nutrient.

By doing so, we can optimize our health and prevent or treat various diseases and conditions that are caused or influenced by nutrient imbalances or deficiencies.

Understanding Nutrient Absorption

Nutrient absorption is the process of transferring nutrients from the food we eat into our bloodstream and cells. It is a crucial step for ensuring that our body gets the nutrients it needs to function properly and stay healthy. However, nutrient absorption is not a simple or uniform process. It is influenced by various factors, such as the type, form, and amount of the nutrient, the presence of other nutrients or substances, the condition of the digestive system, and the individual's genetic makeup.

Nutrient absorption occurs mainly in the small intestine, where the food is broken down into smaller molecules by enzymes and bile. The small intestine has a large surface area, thanks to the presence of finger-like projections called villi and microvilli. These structures increase the contact between the food and the intestinal cells, facilitating the transfer of nutrients into the blood vessels and lymphatic vessels. Some nutrients, such as water and some minerals, can be absorbed by simple diffusion, meaning that they move from an area of high concentration to an area of low concentration. Other nutrients, such as glucose and amino acids, require active transport, meaning that they need energy and carrier proteins to move across the intestinal membrane. Some nutrients, such as fat-soluble vitamins and fatty acids, need to be emulsified by bile and packaged into small droplets called micelles before they can be absorbed.

Nutrient absorption can be enhanced or impaired by various factors, such as the source, form, and dose of the nutrient, the presence of other nutrients or substances, the condition of the digestive system, and the individual's genetic makeup. For example, some nutrients are more bioavailable, meaning that they are more easily absorbed and utilized by the body when they come from animal sources than from plant sources. This is the case for iron, zinc, and vitamin B12. Some nutrients are more bioavailable when they are in certain forms, such as chelated minerals, methylated vitamins, or liquid supplements. Some nutrients can compete with each other for absorption, such as calcium and iron or magnesium and zinc. Some nutrients can enhance or inhibit the absorption of other nutrients, such as vitamin C and iron, or vitamin D and calcium. Some substances, such as fiber, phytates, oxalates, or tannins, can bind to certain nutrients and reduce their absorption. Some conditions, such as inflammation, infection, or disease, can damage the intestinal lining and impair the absorption of nutrients. Some genetic variations, such as mutations or polymorphisms, can affect the expression or function of enzymes or transporters involved in nutrient absorption.

Understanding nutrient absorption is important for optimizing our health and well-being. By knowing how nutrients are absorbed and what factors affect their absorption, we can make better dietary choices and supplement decisions that suit our individual needs and goals. Moreover, nutrient absorption can help us prevent or treat various diseases and conditions that are caused or influenced by nutrient imbalances or deficiencies. For instance, vitamin D, vitamin C, and iodine are three nutrients that play vital roles in our immune system, bone health, and thyroid function, respectively. By ensuring adequate intake and absorption of these nutrients, we can boost our immunity, prevent osteoporosis, and support our metabolism.

CHAPTER 1

DISCOVERING VITAMIN D'S ROLE IN OVERALL HEALTH

Vitamin D is one of the four fat-soluble vitamins, along with vitamins A, E, and K. It is also known as the sunshine vitamin because it can be synthesized by the skin when exposed to ultraviolet rays from the sun. Vitamin D is essential for many aspects of our health, especially for our bones, immune system, and eyes.

Sunshine Vitamin: How Sunlight Impacts Vitamin D Synthesis.

Sunlight exposure is the primary source of vitamin D for humans. When the skin is exposed to ultraviolet B (UVB) rays from the sun, a cholesterol-like molecule called 7-dehydrocholesterol is converted into previtamin D3, which is then transformed into vitamin D3 by the heat of the skin.

Vitamin D3 is then transported to the liver, where it is converted into 25-hydroxyvitamin D (25(OH)D), the main circulating form of vitamin D.

25(OH)D is then transported to the kidneys, where it is converted into 1,25-dihydroxyvitamin D (1,25(OH)2D), the active form of vitamin D that can bind to vitamin D receptors (VDRs) in various tissues and organs.

The amount of vitamin D synthesized by the skin depends on several factors, such as the latitude, season, time of day, cloud cover, air pollution, skin pigmentation, age, clothing, sunscreen use, and genetic variations. Generally, the optimal time for vitamin D synthesis is between 10 a.m. and 3 p.m., when the sun is at its highest point in the sky and the UVB rays are most intense. However, this may vary depending on the location and the season. For example, in regions above 37 degrees north or below 37 degrees south, there is little or no vitamin D synthesis during the winter months due to the low angle and intensity of the sun. Moreover, darker skin tones, older age, and sunscreen use can reduce the amount of vitamin D synthesized by the skin as they block or absorb more UVB rays.

The recommended amount of vitamin D for adults is 600 international units (IU) per day, according to the Institute of Medicine (IOM). However, this may vary depending on the individual's needs and goals. For example, some experts suggest that higher doses of vitamin D may be beneficial for preventing or treating certain diseases and conditions, such as osteoporosis, rickets, multiple sclerosis, diabetes, and depression. However, excessive intake of vitamin D can also cause toxicity, leading to symptoms such as nausea, vomiting, weakness, confusion, kidney stones, and calcification of soft tissues. Therefore, it is important to monitor the blood levels of 25(OH)D and consult a health professional before taking high doses of vitamin D supplements.

Health Benefits Beyond Bone Strength

Vitamin D is best known for its role in bone health, as it helps the body absorb calcium and phosphorus, the two minerals that are essential for building and maintaining strong bones and teeth. Vitamin D deficiency can cause rickets in children, a condition characterized by soft and deformed bones, and osteomalacia in adults, a condition characterized by weak and brittle bones. Vitamin D supplementation can prevent or treat these conditions, as well as osteoporosis, a condition characterized by low bone density and an increased risk of fractures.

However, vitamin D has many other health benefits beyond bone strength, as it is involved in various biological processes, such as immune function, cell growth, inflammation, and hormone regulation. Vitamin D can modulate the activity and expression of various immune cells, such as macrophages, dendritic cells, T cells, and B cells, enhancing the innate immune response and regulating the adaptive immune response. Vitamin D deficiency can impair the immune system and increase the susceptibility to infections, autoimmune diseases, and cancer. Vitamin D supplementation can boost the immune system and protect against these diseases, as well as reduce the severity and duration of respiratory infections such as the common cold and the flu.

Vitamin D can also influence the growth and differentiation of various cells, such as skin cells, hair follicles, and nerve cells, by binding to VDRs and regulating the expression of genes involved in these processes. Vitamin D deficiency can affect the health and appearance of the skin and hair, as well as the function and development of the nervous system. Vitamin D supplementation can improve skin and hair quality, as well as cognitive and mental health, by promoting the production of collagen, keratin, and neurotransmitters such as serotonin and dopamine.

Vitamin D can also modulate the production and action of various hormones, such as insulin, parathyroid hormone, and sex hormones, by interacting with their receptors and enzymes. Vitamin D deficiency can disrupt the hormonal balance and cause various metabolic and reproductive disorders, such as diabetes, obesity, polycystic ovary syndrome, and erectile dysfunction. Vitamin D supplementation can improve the hormonal balance and prevent or treat these disorders, as well as enhance fertility and sexual function, by improving insulin sensitivity, reducing parathyroid hormone levels, and increasing testosterone and estrogen levels.

Vitamin D is a vital nutrient for our health and well-being. It can be obtained from sunlight exposure, supplements, or fortified foods. By ensuring adequate intake and synthesis of vitamin D, we can reap its benefits for our bones, immune system, and eyes, as well as for our skin, hair, nervous system, and hormones.

CHAPTER 2

HARNESSING THE IMMUNE BOOST: THE IMPACT OF VITAMIN C

Vitamin C is one of the eight water-soluble vitamins, along with the B-complex vitamins. It is also known as ascorbic acid because it prevents and cures scurvy, a disease caused by vitamin C deficiency. Vitamin C is essential for many aspects of our health, especially for our immune system, skin, and blood vessels.

Vitamin C and Immune System Function

The body's defense system against pathogens like bacteria, viruses, fungi, and parasites is the immune system. It consists of two main branches: the innate immune system and the adaptive immune system. The innate immune system is the first line of defense, providing a rapid and nonspecific response to any potential threat. The adaptive immune system is the second line of defense, providing a slower but more specific and long-lasting response to a particular antigen.

The immune system relies on various cells, molecules, and organs to perform its functions, such as macrophages, neutrophils, natural killer cells, dendritic cells, mast cells, complement proteins, cytokines, antibodies, T cells, B cells, thymus, spleen, lymph nodes, and bone marrow.

Vitamin C is involved in various aspects of immune system function, such as:

- **Enhancing the production and activity of immune cells:** Vitamin C can stimulate the proliferation and differentiation of various immune cells, such as macrophages, neutrophils, natural killer cells, dendritic cells, mast cells, T cells, and B cells, by acting as a cofactor for enzymes involved in these processes. Vitamin C can also enhance the phagocytic and killing activity of macrophages and neutrophils, the cytotoxic and regulatory activity of natural killer cells and T cells, the antigen-presenting and signaling activity of dendritic cells and mast cells, and the antibody-producing and memory activity of B cells.

- **Protecting the immune cells from oxidative stress:** Vitamin C is a potent antioxidant that can scavenge and neutralize free radicals and reactive oxygen species (ROS) that are generated during the immune response. Free radicals and ROS can damage the DNA, proteins, and membranes of immune cells, impairing their function and survival. Vitamin C can protect the immune cells from oxidative stress by donating electrons to free radicals and ROS, regenerating other antioxidants, such as glutathione and vitamin E, and modulating the way that genes related to antioxidant defense are expressed.

- **Regulating the inflammation and immune response:** Vitamin C can modulate the production and action of various inflammatory and immune mediators, such as cytokines, chemokines, histamine, prostaglandins, and leukotrienes, by influencing their synthesis, degradation, and receptor binding. Vitamin C can also regulate the balance between the pro-inflammatory and anti-inflammatory responses, as well as the balance between the Th1 and Th2 responses, by affecting the polarization and activation of T cells and macrophages. Vitamin C can also influence the expression and function of various transcription factors, such as nuclear factor-kappa B (NF-κB) and activator protein-1 (AP-1), that are involved in the regulation of inflammation and immune responses.

Vitamin C deficiency can impair the immune system and increase the susceptibility to infections, autoimmune diseases, and cancer. Vitamin C supplementation can boost the immune system and protect against these diseases, as well as reduce the severity and duration of respiratory infections such as the common cold and the flu.

Exploring Antioxidant Properties

Vitamin C is not only an essential nutrient for the immune system but also a powerful antioxidant for the whole body. Antioxidants are substances that can prevent or delay the oxidation of other molecules, such as lipids, proteins, and DNA, by free radicals and ROS. Oxidation is a chemical reaction that involves the loss of electrons and can cause cellular damage, aging, and disease.

Free radicals and ROS are unstable and highly reactive molecules that have one or more unpaired electrons and can be generated by various internal and external sources, such as metabolism, inflammation, infection, pollution, smoking, radiation, and stress.

Vitamin C can exert its antioxidant effects by:

- **Scavenging and neutralizing free radicals and ROS:** Vitamin C can donate electrons to free radicals and ROS, such as hydroxyl radicals, superoxide anion, hydrogen peroxide, singlet oxygen, and nitric oxide, and convert them into less reactive or harmless molecules, such as water and dehydroascorbic acid. Vitamin C can also react with metal ions, such as iron and copper, and prevent them from catalyzing the formation of more free radicals and ROS.

- **Regenerating other antioxidants:** Vitamin C can restore the antioxidant capacity of other antioxidants, such as glutathione, vitamin E, and uric acid, by donating electrons to them and reducing them to their active forms. Vitamin C can also recycle itself by being reduced back to ascorbic acid from dehydroascorbic acid by various enzymes and cofactors, such as glutathione, NADPH, and thioredoxin.

- **Modulating the expression of genes involved in antioxidant defense:** Vitamin C can influence the expression and function of various genes that encode for enzymes and proteins involved in antioxidant defense, such as superoxide dismutase, catalase, glutathione peroxidase, glutathione reductase, glutathione S-transferase, heme oxygenase-1, and metallothionein. Vitamin C can also affect the activity and stability of various transcription factors, such as NF-κB, AP-1, and nuclear factor erythroid 2-related factor 2 (Nrf2), that regulate the expression of these genes.

Vitamin C can protect the body from oxidative stress and its consequences, such as cellular damage, aging, and disease. Vitamin C can also enhance the health and function of various tissues and organs that are exposed to high levels of oxidative stress, such as the skin, blood vessels, eyes, brain, heart, and lungs.

CHAPTER 3

IODINE'S CRUCIAL ROLE IN THYROID FUNCTION

Iodine is one of the 16 minerals that are essential for human health. It is also one of the trace elements, meaning that it is needed in very small amounts, usually less than 200 micrograms per day. Iodine is mainly found in the ocean, where it is concentrated by seaweeds and marine animals. Iodine is also added to table salt and some foods, such as dairy products, eggs, and bread, to prevent iodine deficiency. Iodine is essential for the synthesis and function of thyroid hormones, which regulate various aspects of our metabolism, growth, and development.

Thyroid Health Essentials

The thyroid is part of the endocrine system, which consists of various glands that secrete hormones into the bloodstream. The thyroid produces two main hormones: thyroxine (T4) and triiodothyronine (T3), which contain four and three atoms of iodine, respectively.

These hormones are synthesized from the amino acids tyrosine and iodine, which are transported to the thyroid by the blood. The synthesis and secretion of thyroid hormones are regulated by the hypothalamus and the pituitary gland, which are located in the brain. The hypothalamus produces thyrotropin-releasing hormone (TRH), which stimulates the pituitary gland to produce thyroid-stimulating hormone (TSH), which in turn stimulates the thyroid to produce T4 and T3. The levels of thyroid hormones are monitored by a negative feedback loop, meaning that high levels of thyroid hormones inhibit the production of TRH and TSH, and vice versa.

Thyroid hormones have various roles in the body, such as:

- **Regulating the basal metabolic rate (BMR):** Thyroid hormones increase the rate at which the body uses oxygen and energy to perform its basic functions, such as breathing, heartbeat, and digestion. Thyroid hormones also affect the synthesis and breakdown of carbohydrates, fats, and proteins, as well as the production and utilization of glucose and cholesterol.

- **Promoting the growth and development of various tissues and organs:** Thyroid hormones are essential for the normal growth and development of the skeletal system, the nervous system, the reproductive system, and the immune system. Thyroid hormones also influence the expression and function of various growth factors, such as insulin-like growth factor-1 (IGF-1), epidermal growth factor (EGF), and nerve growth factor (NGF).

- **Modulating the activity and sensitivity of other hormones and neurotransmitters:** Thyroid hormones can affect the production and action of various hormones and neurotransmitters, such as adrenaline, cortisol, estrogen, testosterone, serotonin, dopamine, and acetylcholine, by influencing their synthesis, degradation, and receptor binding.

Iodine deficiency or excess can impair the synthesis and function of thyroid hormones and cause various thyroid disorders, such as goiter, hypothyroidism, hyperthyroidism, and thyroid cancer.

Iodine supplementation can prevent or treat these disorders, as well as improve metabolic and cognitive health, by ensuring an adequate and balanced intake of iodine.

Iodine Deficiency and Its Implications

Iodine deficiency is a condition in which the body does not have enough iodine to produce sufficient amounts of thyroid hormones. Iodine deficiency is one of the most common and preventable causes of mental and physical impairment in the world, affecting more than two billion people, especially in developing countries where iodized salt and other sources of iodine are scarce or unavailable. Iodine deficiency can result from various factors, such as low dietary intake of iodine, poor absorption of iodine, high consumption of goitrogens, which are substances that interfere with iodine uptake or utilization, such as cassava, cabbage, broccoli, soy, and millet, and exposure to environmental pollutants, such as perchlorate, which can compete with iodine for transport and uptake.

Iodine deficiency can cause various symptoms and complications, such as:

- **Goiter:** Goiter is an enlargement of the thyroid gland, which occurs as a result of the stimulation of TSH and the accumulation of thyroglobulin, a precursor of thyroid hormones, in the thyroid follicles. Goiter can cause cosmetic and functional problems, such as difficulty breathing, swallowing, and speaking, as well as compression of the trachea, esophagus, and blood vessels.

- **Hypothyroidism:** Hypothyroidism is a condition in which the thyroid gland does not produce enough thyroid hormones, leading to a low BMR and a reduced response to other hormones and neurotransmitters. Hypothyroidism can cause various symptoms, such as fatigue, weight gain, cold intolerance, dry skin, hair loss, constipation, depression, memory loss, and menstrual irregularities.

- **Cretinism:** Cretinism is a severe form of mental and physical retardation that occurs in infants and children who are born to mothers with iodine deficiency during pregnancy. Cretinism can cause various abnormalities, such as stunted growth, delayed development, intellectual disability, deafness, muteness, spasticity, and facial deformities.

- **Thyroid cancer:** Thyroid cancer is a malignant tumor that originates from the thyroid cells. Thyroid cancer can be caused by various factors, such as genetic mutations, radiation exposure, and chronic inflammation. Iodine deficiency can increase the risk of thyroid cancer, especially follicular and anaplastic types, by inducing goiter, hypothyroidism, and oxidative stress. Iodine supplementation can reduce the risk of thyroid cancer, especially papillary and medullary types, by preventing goiter, hypothyroidism, and oxidative stress.

Iodine-Rich Foods:Nourishing The Thyroid Gland

Iodine is a water-soluble mineral that cannot be synthesized or stored by the human body. Therefore, it needs to be obtained from the diet on a regular basis. The recommended dietary intake (RDI) for iodine for adults is 150 micrograms (mcg) per day, according to the IOM. However, this may vary depending on the individual's needs and goals. For example, some experts suggest that higher intakes of iodine may be beneficial for preventing or treating certain thyroid disorders, such as goiter, hypothyroidism, and thyroid cancer. However, excessive intake of iodine can also cause adverse effects, such as hyperthyroidism, autoimmune thyroiditis, and iodine-induced goiter. Therefore, it is important to monitor the intake and urine levels of iodine and consult a health professional before taking high doses of iodine supplements. Iodine can be found in various foods, especially seafood, iodized salt, and seaweed. However, there are many other sources of iodine that are often overlooked or underestimated, such as:

- **Dairy products:** Dairy products, such as milk, cheese, yogurt, and butter, are rich in iodine, as well as other nutrients such as calcium, protein, and vitamin D. The iodine content of dairy products depends on the iodine intake of the cows, the processing methods, and the storage conditions. One cup of milk contains about 50 to 100 mcg of iodine, which is about one-third to two-thirds of the RDI for adults.
- **Eggs:** Eggs are a good source of iodine as well as other nutrients such as protein, choline, and lutein. The iodine content of eggs depends on the iodine intake of the

hens, the feed composition, and the cooking methods. One large egg contains about 20 to 40 mcg of iodine, which is about one-seventh to one-fourth of the RDI for adults.

- **Bread:** Bread is a staple food that is fortified with iodine in many countries, such as the United States, Canada, Australia, and New Zealand. The iodine content of bread depends on the type of flour, the amount of salt, and the baking process. One slice of bread contains about 10 to 60 mcg of iodine, which is about one-fifteenth to two-fifths of the RDI for adults.

- **Prunes:** Prunes are dried plums that are high in iodine, as well as other nutrients such as fiber, potassium, and phenolic compounds. The iodine content of prunes depends on the variety of plums, the drying methods, and the storage conditions. One cup of prunes contains about 10 to 30 mcg of iodine, which is about one-fifteenth to one-fifth of the RDI for adults.

- **Turkey:** Turkey is a lean meat that is rich in iodine as well as other nutrients such as protein, iron, and selenium. The iodine content of turkey depends on the iodine intake of the turkeys, the feed composition, and the cooking methods. One ounce of turkey breast contains about 10 to 20 mcg of iodine, which is about one-fifteenth to one-eighth of the RDI for adults.

Iodine is a vital mineral for the synthesis and function of thyroid hormones, which regulate various aspects of our metabolism, growth, and development. Iodine can be obtained from various foods, especially seafood, iodized salt, and seaweed, as well as dairy products, eggs, bread, prunes, and turkey. By ensuring an adequate and balanced intake of iodine, we can prevent or treat various thyroid disorders, such as goiter, hypothyroidism, hyperthyroidism, and thyroid cancer.

CHAPTER 4

SUNLIGHT AND WELLNESS: A DEEP DIVE INTO VITAMIN D SOURCES

Vitamin D is one of the four fat-soluble vitamins, along with vitamins A, E, and K. It is also known as the sunshine vitamin because it can be synthesized by the skin when exposed to ultraviolet rays from the sun. Vitamin D is essential for many aspects of our health, especially for our bones, immune system, and eyes.

Natural Sun Exposure Guidelines

The main source of vitamin D for humans is sunlight exposure. When the skin is exposed to ultraviolet B (UVB) rays from the sun, a cholesterol-like molecule called 7-dehydrocholesterol is converted into previtamin D3, which is then transformed into vitamin D3 by the heat of the skin. Vitamin D3 is then transported to the liver, where it is converted into 25-hydroxyvitamin D (25(OH)D), the main circulating form of vitamin D. 25(OH)D is then transported to the kidneys, where it is converted into 1,25-dihydroxyvitamin D (1,25(OH)2D), the active form of vitamin D that can bind to vitamin D receptors (VDRs) in various tissues and organs.

The amount of vitamin D synthesized by the skin depends on several factors, such as the latitude, season, time of day, cloud cover, air pollution, skin pigmentation, age, clothing, sunscreen use, and genetic variations. Generally, the optimal time for vitamin D synthesis is between 10 a.m. and 3 p.m., when the sun is at its highest point in the sky and the UVB rays are most intense. However, this may vary depending on the location and the season. For example, in regions above 37 degrees north or below 37 degrees south, there is little or no vitamin D synthesis during the winter months due to the low angle and intensity of the sun. Moreover, darker skin tones, older age, and sunscreen use can reduce the amount of vitamin D synthesized by the skin as they block or absorb more UVB rays.

The recommended amount of vitamin D for adults is 600 international units (IU) per day, according to the Institute of Medicine (IOM). However, this may vary depending on the individual's needs and goals.

For example, some experts suggest that higher doses of vitamin D may be beneficial for preventing or treating certain diseases and conditions, such as osteoporosis, rickets, multiple sclerosis, diabetes, and depression. However, excessive intake of vitamin D can also cause toxicity, leading to symptoms such as nausea, vomiting, weakness, confusion, kidney stones, and calcification of soft tissues. Therefore, it is important to monitor the blood levels of 25(OH)D and consult a health professional before taking high doses of vitamin D supplements.

To obtain the recommended amount of vitamin D from sunlight exposure, the following guidelines can be followed:

- Expose about 40% of the body surface area to the sun for about 15 minutes, two to three times per week, between 10 a.m. and 3 p.m. This can be achieved by wearing shorts and a T-shirt or a swimsuit, depending on the weather and the comfort level. This can provide about 10,000 to 20,000 IU of vitamin D per session, which is more than enough to meet the daily requirement. However, this may vary depending on the factors mentioned above, such as latitude, season, skin tone, and sunscreen use. Therefore, it is advisable to adjust the exposure time and frequency according to the individual's response and preference.

- Avoid sunburn and excessive tanning. Sunburn and excessive tanning are signs of skin damage caused by overexposure to ultraviolet rays, which can increase the risk of skin cancer and premature aging. Moreover, sunburn and excessive tanning can reduce the ability of the skin to synthesize vitamin D, as they increase the production of melanin, a pigment that protects the skin from UV rays but also blocks or absorbs them. Therefore, it is advisable to limit the exposure time to the sun to avoid sunburn and excessive tanning and to apply sunscreen with a sun protection factor (SPF) of at least 15 after the initial exposure time to protect the skin from further damage.

- Consider the individual's health status and medication use: Some health conditions and medications can affect the synthesis and metabolism of vitamin D, as well as the sensitivity to UV rays. For example, people with kidney or liver disease, obesity, malabsorption, or genetic disorders may have impaired conversion of vitamin D to its active form and may require higher doses of vitamin D supplements. People who take certain medications, such as anticonvulsants, corticosteroids, or antiretrovirals, may have reduced levels of vitamin D and may require higher doses of vitamin D supplements. People who have skin conditions, such as psoriasis, eczema, or lupus, may have increased sensitivity to UV rays and may require a lower exposure time to the sun or avoid it altogether. Therefore, it is advisable to consult a health professional before exposing yourself to the sun and to follow their recommendations regarding the appropriate exposure time, frequency, and supplementation.

Sunlight exposure is a natural and effective way to obtain vitamin D, as well as to enjoy the benefits of the sun for our mood, circadian rhythm, and overall well-being. By following the guidelines above, we can optimize our vitamin D synthesis and avoid the risks of deficiency or toxicity, as well as the risks of skin damage or cancer.

Supplements and Fortified Foods

Sunlight exposure is the main source of vitamin D for humans, but it may not be sufficient or feasible for everyone due to various factors, such as latitude, season, weather, lifestyle, health status, and personal preference. Therefore, other sources of vitamin D, such as supplements and fortified foods, may be needed or preferred to meet the daily requirement and prevent or treat deficiency.

Supplements are products that contain concentrated amounts of nutrients, such as vitamins, minerals, amino acids, fatty acids, and herbs, that are intended to supplement the diet and provide additional health benefits. Supplements can be found in various forms, such as tablets, capsules, liquids, powders, or gummies, and can be purchased from pharmacies, health food stores, or online retailers.

Supplements can be useful for people who have difficulty obtaining enough nutrients from their diet due to various reasons, such as food allergies, intolerances, preferences, or restrictions, or who have increased needs for certain nutrients due to various reasons, such as pregnancy, lactation, aging, illness, or medication use.

Fortified foods are foods that have been enriched with nutrients that are not naturally present or are present in insufficient amounts to improve their nutritional value and prevent or treat deficiency. Fortification can be done by adding synthetic or natural forms of nutrients to the food during processing or by spraying or coating the food with nutrients after processing. Fortification can be mandatory or voluntary, depending on the regulations and policies of each country or region. Fortified foods can be beneficial for people who have limited access to or exposure to natural sources of nutrients due to various reasons, such as poverty, geography, or culture, or who have low intake or absorption of certain nutrients due to various reasons, such as poor appetite, digestion, or absorption.

Vitamin D supplements and fortified foods can provide an alternative or additional source of vitamin D, especially for people who have low or no sunlight exposure or who have increased needs or risks for deficiency.

However, there are some considerations and precautions that need to be taken into account when choosing and using these sources, such as:

- **The type, form, and dose of vitamin D:** There are two main types of vitamin D that are used in supplements and fortified foods: vitamin D2 (ergocalciferol) and vitamin D3 (cholecalciferol). Vitamin D2 is derived from plant sources, such as mushrooms or yeast, while vitamin D3 is derived from animal sources, such as lanolin or fish oil. Both types of vitamin D can raise the blood levels of 25(OH)D, but vitamin D3 is more potent and effective than vitamin D2, as it is more similar to the vitamin D synthesized by the skin. Therefore, vitamin D3 is preferred over vitamin D2 for supplementation and fortification. Vitamin D can also be found in various forms, such as tablets, capsules, liquids, powders, or gummies, and can be combined with other nutrients, such as calcium, magnesium, or zinc. The form of vitamin D may affect its absorption and bioavailability, as well as its convenience and palatability. Generally, liquid and powder forms of vitamin D are more easily absorbed and utilized by the body than tablet and capsule forms, as they do not need to be broken down by the digestive system. However, liquid and powder forms of vitamin D may also be more prone to degradation and contamination than tablet and capsule forms, as they are more exposed to light, heat, and moisture. Therefore, the form of vitamin D should be chosen according to the individual's preferences and needs. The dose of vitamin D may vary depending on the individual's age, weight, health status, and goals. The RDA for vitamin D for adults is 600 IU per day, according to the IOM. However, some experts suggest that higher doses of vitamin D may be beneficial for preventing or treating certain diseases and conditions, such as osteoporosis, rickets, multiple sclerosis, diabetes, and depression. However, excessive intake of vitamin D can also cause toxicity, leading to symptoms such as nausea, vomiting, weakness, confusion, kidney stones, and calcification of soft tissues.

Therefore, the dose of vitamin D should be chosen according to the individual's needs and goals and monitored by the blood levels of 25(OH)D and the symptoms of deficiency or toxicity.

- **The quality, safety, and efficacy of vitamin D:** Not all supplements and fortified foods are created equal, and some may contain more or less vitamin D than what is stated on the label or may contain contaminants or additives that may affect the quality, safety, and efficacy of vitamin D. Therefore, it is advisable to choose reputable brands and products that have been tested and certified by independent third-party organizations, such as the United States Pharmacopeia (USP), the

National Sanitation Foundation (NSF), or ConsumerLab.com, and to follow the instructions and precautions on the label and the package insert.

- **The interactions and side effects of vitamin D:** Vitamin D can interact with other nutrients, medications, or supplements and cause adverse effects or reduce their effectiveness. For example, vitamin D can enhance the absorption of calcium and phosphorus but also increase the risk of hypercalcemia and kidney stones, especially if taken with high doses of calcium or phosphorus supplements. Vitamin D can also interfere with the metabolism of certain medications, such as anticonvulsants, corticosteroids, or antiretrovirals, reduce their blood levels and efficacy, or increase their side effects. Therefore, it is advisable to consult a health professional before taking vitamin D supplements, to inform them of any other nutrients, medications, or supplements that are being taken, and to monitor the blood levels and the symptoms of vitamin D and the other substances.

Supplements and fortified foods can provide an alternative or additional source of vitamin D, especially for people who have low or no sunlight exposure or who have increased needs or risks for deficiency. However, there are some considerations and precautions that need to be taken into account when choosing and using these sources, such as the type, form, dose, quality, safety, efficacy, interactions, and side effects of vitamin D. By following these guidelines, we can optimize our vitamin D intake and avoid the risks of deficiency or toxicity, as well as the risks of interactions or side effects.

CHAPTER 5

BEYOND ORANGES: DIVERSE SOURCES OF VITAMIN C FOR OPTIMAL HEALTH

Vitamin C is one of the eight water-soluble vitamins, along with the B-complex vitamins. It is also known as ascorbic acid because it prevents and cures scurvy, a disease caused by vitamin C deficiency. Vitamin C is essential for many aspects of our health, especially for our immune system, skin, and blood vessels.

Vitamin C and Its Functions in the Body

Vitamin C is involved in various functions in the body, such as:

- **Enhancing the production and activity of immune cells:** Vitamin C can stimulate the proliferation and differentiation of various immune cells, such as macrophages, neutrophils, natural killer cells, dendritic cells, mast cells, T cells, and B cells, by acting as a cofactor for enzymes involved in these processes. Vitamin C can also enhance the phagocytic and killing activity of macrophages and neutrophils, the cytotoxic and regulatory activity of natural killer cells and T cells, the antigen-presenting and signaling activity of dendritic cells and mast cells, and the antibody-producing and memory activity of B cells.

- **Protecting the immune cells from oxidative stress:** Vitamin C is a potent antioxidant that can scavenge and neutralize free radicals and reactive oxygen species (ROS) that are generated during the immune response. Free radicals and ROS can damage the DNA, proteins, and membranes of immune cells, impairing their function and survival. Vitamin C can protect the immune cells from oxidative stress by donating electrons to free radicals and ROS, regenerating other antioxidants such as glutathione and vitamin E.

- **Regulating the inflammation and immune response:** Vitamin C can modulate the production and action of various inflammatory and immune mediators, such as cytokines, chemokines, histamine, prostaglandins, and leukotrienes, by influencing their synthesis, degradation, and receptor binding. Vitamin C can also regulate the balance between the pro-inflammatory and anti-inflammatory responses, as well as the balance between the Th1 and Th2 responses, by affecting the polarization and activation of T cells and macrophages. Vitamin C can also influence the expression and function of various transcription factors, such as nuclear factor-kappa B (NF-κB) and activator protein-1 (AP-1), that are involved in the regulation of inflammation and immune responses.

- **Supporting the Synthesis and Maintenance of Collagen:** Collagen is the most abundant protein in the body and the main component of connective tissues such as skin, bones, cartilage, tendons, ligaments, and blood vessels. Collagen provides strength, elasticity, and structure to these tissues and also facilitates wound healing and tissue repair. Vitamin C is required for the synthesis of collagen, as it acts as a cofactor for the enzymes that hydroxylate proline and lysine, the amino acids that are essential for the stability and cross-linking of collagen fibers. Vitamin C also protects collagen from degradation by free radicals and ROS and stimulates the production of other proteins and molecules that are involved in collagen synthesis and maturation, such as elastin, fibronectin, and hyaluronic acid.

- **Enhancing the absorption and utilization of iron:** Iron is a mineral that is essential for the production of hemoglobin, the protein that carries oxygen in the red blood cells, and myoglobin, the protein that stores oxygen in the muscle cells. Iron is also involved in various enzymatic reactions, such as the synthesis of DNA, RNA, and neurotransmitters. Iron can be found in two forms in food: heme iron and non-heme iron. Heme iron is derived from animal sources, such as meat, poultry, and fish, and is more easily absorbed and utilized by the body than non-heme iron. Non-heme iron is derived from plant sources, such as beans, lentils, nuts, seeds, and grains, and is less easily absorbed and utilized by the body than heme iron. Vitamin C can enhance the absorption and utilization of non-heme iron by reducing it from the ferric form (Fe^{3+}) to the ferrous form (Fe^{2+}), which is more soluble and bioavailable, and by forming complexes with iron that can prevent its binding to inhibitors, such as phytates, oxalates, and polyphenols, that are present in plant foods.

Vitamin C deficiency can impair the functions of vitamin C in the body and cause various symptoms and complications, such as scurvy, infections, bleeding gums, bruising, poor wound healing, anemia, and fatigue. Vitamin C supplementation can prevent or treat these conditions, as well as improve the immune system, skin, and blood vessel health, by ensuring an adequate and balanced intake of vitamin C.

Diverse Sources of Vitamin C for Optimal Health

Vitamin C is a water-soluble vitamin that cannot be synthesized or stored by the human body. Therefore, it needs to be obtained from the diet on a regular basis. The recommended dietary allowance (RDA) for vitamin C for adults is 90 milligrams (mg) per day for men and 75 mg per day for women, according to the IOM. However, this may vary depending on the individual's needs and goals.

For example, some experts suggest that higher doses of vitamin C may be beneficial for preventing or treating certain diseases and conditions, such as scurvy, infections, allergies, asthma, and cancer. However, excessive intake of vitamin C can also cause adverse effects, such as diarrhea, nausea, abdominal cramps, kidney stones, and iron overload. Therefore, it is important to monitor the intake and blood levels of vitamin C and consult a health professional before taking high doses of vitamin C supplements. Vitamin C can be found in various fruits and vegetables, especially citrus fruits, such as oranges, lemons, grapefruits, and limes. However, there are many other sources of vitamin C that are often overlooked or underestimated, such as:

- **Bell peppers:** Bell peppers, especially red ones, are rich in vitamin C as well as other antioxidants, such as beta-carotene, lutein, and zeaxanthin. One cup of raw red bell pepper contains about 190 mg of vitamin C, which is more than twice the RDA for adults.

- **Broccoli:** Broccoli is a cruciferous vegetable that is high in vitamin C as well as other nutrients such as fiber, folate, and sulforaphane. One cup of cooked broccoli contains about 100 mg of vitamin C, which is more than the RDA for adults.

- **Strawberries:** Strawberries are a delicious and nutritious fruit that are loaded with vitamin C as well as other phytochemicals, such as anthocyanins, flavonoids, and ellagic acid. One cup of sliced strawberries contains about 90 mg of vitamin C, which is almost the RDA for adults.

- **Kiwifruit:** Kiwifruit is a tropical fruit that is packed with vitamin C as well as other vitamins and minerals, such as vitamin K, potassium, and copper. One medium kiwifruit contains about 70 mg of vitamin C, which is almost the RDA for adults.

- **Papaya:** Papaya is a tropical fruit that is rich in vitamin C as well as other enzymes and antioxidants, such as papain, lycopene, and beta-carotene. One cup of cubed papaya contains about 90 mg of vitamin C, which is almost the RDA for adults.

CHAPTER 6

IODINE-RICH FOODS: NOURISHING THE THYROID GLAND

Iodine is an essential trace element that plays a crucial role in thyroid function. The thyroid gland produces hormones that regulate many aspects of metabolism, growth, and development. Iodine is needed for the synthesis of these hormones, namely thyroxine (T4) and triiodothyronine (T3).

Iodine deficiency is a common problem worldwide, affecting more than two billion people. It can cause various health issues, such as goiter (enlarged thyroid gland), hypothyroidism (low thyroid hormone levels), cretinism (severe mental and physical retardation in children), and an increased risk of thyroid cancer. Therefore, it is important to ensure adequate iodine intake from dietary sources or supplements.

In this chapter, we will explore some of the best foods that provide iodine and how to incorporate them into your diet. We will also discuss some plant-based iodine sources and how to avoid potential iodine toxicity.

Incorporating Seafood Into your Diet

Seafood is the richest natural source of iodine, as marine animals accumulate iodine from seawater and seaweed. Some of the most iodine-dense seafood include:

- **Seaweed:** Seaweed, such as kelp, nori, wakame, and kombu, is a staple food in many Asian cuisines. It can provide up to 2,984 micrograms (mcg) of iodine per gram, which is more than 1,000 times the recommended daily intake (RDI) of 150 mcg. However, the iodine content of seaweed can vary widely depending on the type, origin, season, and preparation method. Therefore, it is advisable to consume seaweed in moderation and check the nutrition label for iodine content, if available. You can eat seaweed powdered, dried, cooked, or uncooked. It can be added to salads, soups, sushi, noodles, or smoothies.

- **Cod:** Cod is a lean, white fish that can provide 99 mcg of iodine per 3-ounce (85-gram) serving, which is 66% of the RDI. Cod is also a good source of protein, vitamin B12, selenium, and phosphorus. Cod can be baked, grilled, fried, or poached. It can be served with lemon, herbs, butter, or sauces.

- **Shrimp:** Shrimp is a type of shellfish that can provide 35 mcg of iodine per 3-ounce (85-gram) serving, which is 23% of the RDI. Shrimp is also rich in protein, selenium, choline, and vitamin B12. Shrimp can be boiled, steamed, roasted, or sautéed. It can be eaten as an appetizer, a salad, or a main dish.

- **Tuna:** Tuna is a fatty, oily fish that can provide 17 mcg of iodine per 3-ounce (85-gram) serving, which is 11% of the RDI. Tuna is also high in protein, omega-3 fatty acids, vitamin D, and selenium. Tuna can be eaten fresh, canned, or frozen. It can be made into sandwiches, salads, casseroles, or sushi.

- **Other seafood:** Other seafood that can provide iodine include salmon, sardines, scallops, lobster, oysters, mussels, and clams. The iodine content of these seafoods can range from 4 to 36 mcg per 3-ounce (85-gram) serving. These seafoods are also nutritious and delicious and can be prepared in various ways.

Seafood is a great way to boost your iodine intake as well as your overall health. However, some people may have allergies, intolerances, or ethical concerns about consuming seafood. In that case, there are other plant-based sources of iodine that can also help meet your needs.

Plant-Based Iodine Sources

Plant-based sources of iodine are generally less reliable than seafood, as the iodine content of plants depends on soil quality, irrigation, and fertilization methods. However, some plants can still provide significant amounts of iodine, especially if they are grown in iodine-rich regions or supplemented with iodine. Some of the plant-based iodine sources include:

- **Iodized salt:** Iodized salt is table salt that has been enhanced with iodine. It is one of the most widely available and affordable sources of iodine, especially in regions where iodine deficiency is prevalent. One teaspoon (5 grams) of iodized salt can provide 76 mcg of iodine, which is 51% of the RDI. However, iodized salt can also contribute to excess sodium intake, which can raise blood pressure and increase the risk of cardiovascular diseases. Therefore, it is advisable to use iodized salt sparingly and choose other sources of iodine whenever possible.

- **Dairy products:** Dairy products, such as milk, cheese, yogurt, and butter, can provide iodine, as cows are often fed with iodine-supplemented feed or salt. The iodine content of dairy products can vary depending on the type, brand, and origin of the product. However, on average, one cup (240 ml) of milk can provide 56 mcg of iodine, which is 37% of the RDI. Dairy products are also good sources of protein, calcium, phosphorus, and vitamin B12. Dairy products can be consumed as beverages, snacks, or ingredients in various dishes.

- **Eggs:** Eggs can provide iodine, as chickens are also often fed with iodine-supplemented feed or salt. The iodine content of eggs can vary depending on the type, brand, and origin of the eggs. However, on average, one large egg can provide 24 mcg of iodine, which is 16% of the RDI. Eggs are also rich in protein, choline, selenium, and vitamin B12. Eggs can be boiled, scrambled, fried, or poached. You can have them for lunch, supper, or breakfast

- **Fruits and vegetables:** Fruits and vegetables can provide iodine, as they absorb iodine from the soil or water. However, the iodine content of fruits and vegetables can vary widely depending on the type, origin, season, and cultivation method of the produce. Some of the fruits and vegetables that can provide iodine include strawberries, cranberries, bananas, prunes, potatoes, green beans, spinach, and lettuce. The iodine content of these fruits and vegetables can range from 2 to 13 mcg per 100 grams. Fruits and vegetables are also excellent sources of fiber, antioxidants, vitamins, and minerals. Fruits and vegetables can be eaten raw, cooked, juiced, or blended.

- **Nuts and seeds:** Nuts and seeds can provide iodine, as they also absorb iodine from the soil or water. However, the iodine content of nuts and seeds can also vary widely depending on the type, origin, season, and cultivation method of the nuts and seeds. Some of the nuts and seeds that can provide iodine include chia seeds, flaxseeds, sunflower seeds, almonds, walnuts, and pistachios. The iodine content of these nuts and seeds can range from 1 to 12 mcg per 100 grams. Nuts and seeds are also great sources of healthy fats, protein, fiber, and minerals. Nuts and seeds can be eaten as snacks, toppings, or ingredients in various dishes.

Plant-based sources of iodine can help you meet your iodine needs as well as provide other health benefits. However, some plant-based sources of iodine may also contain substances that can interfere with iodine absorption or thyroid function, such as goitrogens and thiocyanates. These substances are found in cruciferous vegetables (such as broccoli, cabbage, cauliflower, kale, and Brussels sprouts), soy products (such as tofu, tempeh, soy milk, and soy sauce), and millet. These foods are not necessarily bad for you, but they should be consumed in moderation and preferably cooked, as cooking can reduce their goitrogenic and thiocyanate content.

Avoiding Iodine Toxicity

While iodine is essential for thyroid function and overall health, too much iodine can also be harmful. Excess iodine intake can cause iodine toxicity, which can lead to symptoms such as nausea, vomiting, diarrhea, abdominal pain, fever, headache, metallic taste, and swelling of the salivary glands. In some cases, iodine toxicity can also cause thyroid dysfunction, such as hyperthyroidism (high thyroid hormone levels) or hypothyroidism (low thyroid hormone levels).

The tolerable upper intake level (UL) for iodine is 1,100 mcg per day for adults. This is the maximum amount of iodine that is unlikely to cause adverse health effects. However, some people may be more sensitive to iodine and experience negative effects at lower doses. Therefore, it is advisable to monitor your iodine intake and avoid consuming excessive amounts of iodine from food, supplements, or medications.

Some of the sources of iodine that can cause iodine toxicity include:

- **Seaweed:** As mentioned earlier, seaweed is the richest natural source of iodine, but it can also contain extremely high amounts of iodine that can exceed the UL. For example, one gram of kelp can provide up to 2,984 mcg of iodine, which is more than twice the UL. Therefore, it is important to consume seaweed in moderation and check the nutrition label for iodine content, if available. Seaweed can also contain heavy metals, such as arsenic, mercury, and cadmium, that can pose health risks if consumed in large quantities. Therefore, it is advisable to choose seaweed from reputable sources and limit your intake to no more than two servings per week.

- **Iodine supplements:** Iodine supplements are often used to prevent or treat iodine deficiency, especially in regions where iodine is scarce in the diet. However, iodine supplements can also provide excessive amounts of iodine, which can cause iodine toxicity. For example, one tablet of potassium iodide can provide 130 mg of iodine, which is more than 100 times the UL. Therefore, it is important to consult your doctor before taking any iodine supplements and follow the dosage instructions carefully. Iodine supplements should only be used under medical supervision and for a short period of time.

- **Iodine-containing medications:** Some medications can contain iodine, either as an active ingredient or as an excipient (inactive ingredient). For example, some antiseptics, contrast agents, expectorants, and antiarrhythmics can contain iodine. These medications can also provide excessive amounts of iodine that can cause iodine toxicity. Therefore, it is important to inform your doctor about any medications you are taking and check the label for iodine content, 8if available. You should also avoid taking these medications for a long time or in combination with other sources of iodine.

Iodine toxicity is a rare but serious condition that can affect your thyroid function and overall health. Therefore, it is important to avoid consuming too much iodine from food, supplements, or medications. You should also be aware of the signs and symptoms of iodine toxicity and seek medical attention if you experience any of them. The best way to ensure optimal iodine intake is to eat a balanced diet that includes a variety of iodine-rich foods, such as seafood, dairy products, eggs, fruits, vegetables, nuts, and seeds. You should also use iodized salt sparingly and only take iodine supplements or medications as prescribed by your doctor. By doing so, you can nourish your thyroid gland and enjoy the benefits of iodine for your health and wellness.

CHAPTER 7
THE SCIENCE OF ABSORPTION: OPTIMIZING NUTRIENT UPTAKE

Nutrient uptake is the process of transferring nutrients from the external environment into the internal environment of the body. Nutrient absorption is the process of moving nutrients from the digestive tract into the bloodstream or lymphatic system. Nutrient transport is the process of delivering nutrients to the cells and tissues that need them. These three processes are essential for maintaining health and wellness, as they provide the body with the energy and building blocks it needs to function properly.

However, not all nutrients are equally absorbed and transported by the body. Some nutrients are more bioavailable than others, meaning that they are more readily absorbed and utilized by the body. Some factors that can affect nutrient bioavailability include:

- **The chemical form of the nutrient:** Some nutrients exist in different forms that have different absorption rates and biological activities. For example, iron can be found in two forms: heme iron and non-heme iron. Heme iron is derived from animal sources, such as meat, poultry, and fish. Non-heme iron is derived from plant sources, such as beans, grains, and vegetables. Heme iron is more bioavailable than non-heme iron, as it is more easily absorbed and used by the body. Similarly, vitamin A can be found in two forms: retinol and beta-carotene. Retinol is the active form of vitamin A that is derived from animal sources, such as liver, eggs, and dairy products. Beta-carotene is a precursor of vitamin A that is derived from plant sources, such as carrots, sweet potatoes, and spinach. Beta-carotene has to be converted into retinol by the body before it can be used, which reduces its bioavailability.

- **The presence of other nutrients or substances:** Some nutrients or substances can enhance or inhibit the absorption of other nutrients. For example, vitamin C can enhance the absorption of non-heme iron, as it reduces iron to a more soluble form and forms a complex with it that facilitates its uptake. On the other hand, phytates, oxalates, and polyphenols can inhibit the absorption of non-heme iron, as they bind to iron and form insoluble complexes that prevent its uptake. Similarly, fat-soluble vitamins (A, D, E, and K) require the presence of dietary fat to be absorbed, as they are incorporated into micelles (small droplets of fat) that facilitate their transport across the intestinal wall. On the other hand, fiber can reduce the absorption of fat-soluble vitamins, as it binds to fat and prevents its digestion and absorption.

- **The physiological state of the individual:** Some physiological factors can affect the absorption and transport of nutrients, such as age, health status, genetic variations, and hormonal levels. For example, infants and elderly people have lower gastric acid secretion, which can impair the absorption of some nutrients, such as calcium, iron, and vitamin B12. People with certain diseases or conditions, such as inflammatory bowel disease, celiac disease, or gastric bypass surgery, can have reduced intestinal surface area, which can impair the absorption of most nutrients. People with certain genetic variations, such as mutations in the MTHFR gene, can have impaired metabolism of folate, which can affect the synthesis of DNA and other molecules. People with different hormonal levels, such as pregnant or lactating women, can have increased or decreased requirements for some nutrients, such as iron, calcium, and iodine.

In this chapter, we will explore some of the ways to optimize nutrient uptake, absorption, and transport by considering the factors mentioned above. We will also discuss some of the consequences of nutrient deficiencies and excesses and how to prevent or treat them. By understanding the science of absorption, we can make better dietary choices and improve our health and wellness.

Factors Influencing Nutrient Absorption

As we have seen, nutrient absorption is influenced by various factors, such as the chemical form of the nutrient, the presence of other nutrients or substances, and the physiological state of the individual. In this section, we will examine some of these factors in more detail and provide some practical tips on how to enhance or avoid them.

The Chemical Form of the Nutrient

The chemical form of the nutrient can affect its bioavailability, as different forms have different absorption rates and biological activities. Some nutrients can be found in different forms in food, while others can be modified by the body or by external agents. Some examples of nutrients that have different chemical forms include:

- **Iron:** Heme iron and non-heme iron are the two types of iron. Heme iron is derived from animal sources, such as meat, poultry, and fish. Non-heme iron is derived from plant sources, such as beans, grains, and vegetables. Heme iron is more bioavailable than non-heme iron, as it is more easily absorbed and used by the body. Non-heme iron can also be converted into heme iron by the body, but this process is inefficient and depends on the availability of other nutrients, such as vitamin C. The recommended dietary allowance (RDA) for iron is 8 mg per day for men and postmenopausal women, and 18 mg per day for premenopausal women. However, these values are based on the assumption that only 10% of dietary iron is absorbed, which reflects the average intake of a mixed diet of animal and plant sources. If the diet is predominantly plant-based, the absorption rate may be lower, and the RDA may need to be increased by 1.8 times. To enhance the absorption of non-heme iron, it is advisable to consume it with foods rich in vitamin C, such as citrus fruits, tomatoes, peppers, or broccoli. To avoid the inhibition of non-heme iron absorption, it is advisable to limit the intake of foods rich in phytates, oxalates, and polyphenols, such as whole grains, legumes, nuts, seeds, spinach, rhubarb, tea, and coffee.

- **Vitamin A:** Vitamin A can be found in two forms: retinol and beta-carotene. Retinol is the active form of vitamin A that is derived from animal sources, such as liver, eggs, and dairy products. Beta-carotene is a precursor of vitamin A that is derived from plant sources, such as carrots, sweet potatoes, and spinach. Beta-carotene has to be converted into retinol by the body before it can be used, which reduces its bioavailability. The conversion rate of beta-carotene to retinol depends on several factors, such as the amount and type of beta-carotene, the presence of other carotenoids, the intake of fat and protein, and the physiological state of the individual. On average, it is estimated that 12 mcg of beta-carotene can provide 1 mcg of retinol. The RDA for vitamin A is 900 mcg for men and 700 mcg for women. To enhance the absorption of beta-carotene, it is advisable to consume it with foods rich in fat, such as oil, butter, or cheese. To avoid the inhibition of beta-carotene absorption, it is advisable to limit the intake of foods rich in fiber, such as whole grains, legumes, fruits, and vegetables.

The Presence of Other Nutrients or Substances

The presence of other nutrients or substances can enhance or inhibit the absorption of other nutrients. Some nutrients or substances can act as synergists, meaning that they increase the bioavailability of other nutrients. Some nutrients or substances can act as antagonists, meaning that they decrease the bioavailability of other nutrients. Some examples of nutrients or substances that have synergistic or antagonistic effects include:

- **Vitamin C and iron:** Vitamin C can enhance the absorption of non-heme iron, as it reduces iron to a more soluble form and forms a complex with it that facilitates its uptake. Vitamin C can also prevent the oxidation of iron, which can impair its absorption. Therefore, it is advisable to consume foods rich in vitamin C, such as citrus fruits, tomatoes, peppers, or broccoli, along with foods rich in non-heme iron, such as beans, grains, and vegetables. The recommended dietary intake (RDI) for vitamin C is 90 mg for men and 75 mg for women. However, these values are based on the assumption that only 10% of dietary vitamin C is absorbed, which reflects the average intake of a mixed diet of animal and plant sources. If the diet is predominantly plant-based, the absorption rate may be higher, and the RDI may need to be adjusted accordingly.

- **Phytates, oxalates, polyphenols, and iron:** Phytates, oxalates, and polyphenols can inhibit the absorption of non-heme iron as they bind to it and form insoluble complexes that prevent its uptake. Phytates are found in whole grains, legumes, nuts, and seeds. Oxalates are found in spinach, rhubarb, beet greens, and chocolate. Polyphenols are found in tea, coffee, wine, and cocoa. Therefore, it is advisable to limit the intake of foods rich in phytates, oxalates, and polyphenols, or consume them at different times than foods rich in non-heme iron. Alternatively, the inhibitory effects of these substances can be reduced by soaking, sprouting, fermenting, or cooking the foods that contain them, or by adding foods rich in vitamin C, calcium, or animal protein to the meal.

- **Fat and fat-soluble vitamins:** Fat-soluble vitamins (A, D, E, and K) require the presence of dietary fat to be absorbed, as they are incorporated into micelles (small droplets of fat) that facilitate their transport across the intestinal wall. Therefore, it is advisable to consume foods rich in fat-soluble vitamins, such as liver, eggs, dairy products, carrots, sweet potatoes, and spinach, along with foods rich in fat, such as oil, butter, cheese, or nuts. The RDA for fat-soluble vitamins varies depending on the type and age of the individual. However, these values are based on the assumption that the average intake of dietary fat is 30% of total energy intake, which reflects the typical Western diet. If the diet is low in fat, the absorption rate of fat-soluble vitamins may be lower, and the RDA may need to be increased accordingly.

- **Fiber and fat-soluble vitamins:** Fiber can reduce the absorption of fat-soluble vitamins, as it binds to fat and prevents its digestion and absorption. Fiber is found in whole grains, legumes, fruits, and vegetables.

Therefore, it is advisable to limit the intake of foods rich in fiber or consume them at different times than foods rich in fat-soluble vitamins. Alternatively, the inhibitory effects of fiber can be reduced by adding foods rich in fat, such as oil, butter, cheese, or nuts, to the meal. Fiber is also beneficial for health, as it can lower cholesterol, blood sugar, and blood pressure and promote bowel regularity and satiety. The RDA for fiber is 38 grams for men and 25 grams for women. However, these values are based on the assumption that the average intake of dietary fiber is 15 grams per day, which reflects the typical Western diet. If the diet is high in fiber, the absorption rate of fat-soluble vitamins may be higher, and the RDA may need to be adjusted accordingly.

The Physiological State of the Individual

The physiological state of the individual can affect the absorption and transport of nutrients, such as age, health status, genetic variations, and hormonal levels. Some physiological factors can increase or decrease the requirements for some nutrients, while others can impair or enhance the metabolism of some nutrients. Some examples of physiological factors that can influence nutrient bioavailability include:

- **Age:** Age can affect the absorption and transport of nutrients, as the digestive system and the metabolic pathways change over time. For example, infants and elderly people have lower gastric acid secretion, which can impair the absorption of some nutrients, such as calcium, iron, and vitamin B12. Infants and elderly people also have lower enzyme activity, which can impair the digestion and metabolism of some nutrients, such as lactose, protein, and fat. Therefore, it is advisable to provide infants and elderly people with foods that are easy to digest and absorb, such as breast milk, formula, yogurt, eggs, and fish. Infants and elderly people also have different nutrient requirements than adults, as they have different growth and maintenance needs. Therefore, it is advisable to follow the specific dietary guidelines and recommendations for infants and elderly people, such as the Dietary Reference Intakes (DRIs) and the Dietary Guidelines for Americans (DGAs).

- **Health status:** Health status can affect the absorption and transport of nutrients, as some diseases or conditions can alter the function of the digestive system and the metabolic pathways. For example, people with inflammatory bowel disease, celiac disease, or gastric bypass surgery can have reduced intestinal surface area, which can impair the absorption of most nutrients. People with diabetes, kidney disease, or liver disease can have impaired glucose, protein, or fat metabolism, which can affect the utilization of some nutrients. Therefore, it is advisable to consult a doctor or a dietitian before making any dietary changes, as some foods or supplements may be beneficial or harmful for certain health conditions. People with certain diseases or conditions may also need to follow specific dietary plans or restrictions, such as low-carbohydrate, low-protein, or low-fat diets, to manage their symptoms and complications.

- **Genetic variation:** Genetic variations can affect the absorption and transport of nutrients, as some genes can encode for enzymes, transporters, receptors, or regulators that are involved in the metabolism of some nutrients. For example, people with mutations in the MTHFR gene can have impaired metabolism of folate, which can affect the synthesis of DNA and other molecules. People with mutations in the SLC23A1 gene can have impaired transport of vitamin C, which can affect the synthesis of collagen and other molecules. Therefore, it is advisable to be aware of your genetic profile and how it may affect your nutrient needs and responses. You can obtain your genetic information from a genetic testing service or a health care provider. You can also use online tools or databases, such as

SNPedia, to learn more about your genetic variations and their implications for your health and nutrition.

- **Hormonal levels:** Hormonal levels can affect the absorption and transport of nutrients, as some hormones can regulate the expression or activity of enzymes, transporters, receptors, or regulators that are involved in the metabolism of some nutrients. For example, estrogen and progesterone can affect the metabolism of calcium, magnesium, and vitamin D, which can affect bone health and density. Thyroid hormones can affect the metabolism of iodine, selenium, and zinc, which can affect thyroid function and development. Therefore, it is advisable to monitor your hormonal levels and how they may affect your nutrient needs and responses. You can measure your hormonal levels with a blood test or a saliva test, or use online tools or calculators, such as the Hormone Balance Test, to assess your hormonal balance and health. You can also use natural or synthetic hormones, such as birth control pills, hormone replacement therapy, or supplements, to modulate your hormonal levels and improve your health and wellness. However, you should consult your doctor before using any hormones, as they may have side effects or interactions with other medications or supplements.

Enhancing Bioavailability through Dietary Choices

As we have seen, nutrient bioavailability is influenced by various factors, such as the chemical form of the nutrient, the presence of other nutrients or substances, and the physiological state of the individual. However, we can also enhance the bioavailability of some nutrients by making smart dietary choices and following some simple tips. In this section, we will provide some practical advice on how to optimize nutrient uptake, absorption, and transport by considering the factors mentioned above. Here are some tips to enhance nutrient bioavailability:

- **Eat a balanced and varied diet:** Eating a balanced and varied diet is the best way to ensure optimal nutrient intake and bioavailability, as it provides the body with a wide range of nutrients and substances that can work together to support health and wellness. A balanced and varied diet should include foods from all the major food groups, such as grains, fruits, vegetables, protein, dairy, and fats. A balanced and varied diet should also include foods from different sources, such as animal and plant sources, as they can provide different forms and amounts of nutrients. A balanced and varied diet should also include foods of different colors, flavors, and textures, as they can provide different phytochemicals and antioxidants that can enhance the function and protection of the body. A balanced and varied diet can be achieved by following the Dietary Guidelines for Americans (DGAs), which provide science-based recommendations on what and how much to eat for different age groups, genders, and health conditions.

- **Eat foods in their natural or minimally processed forms:** Eating foods in their natural or minimally processed forms can enhance the bioavailability of some nutrients, as they can preserve the integrity and quality of the nutrients and substances. Natural or minimally processed foods are foods that are obtained directly from nature or undergo little or no alteration before consumption, such as fresh fruits, vegetables, nuts, seeds, eggs, and meat. Natural or minimally processed foods can also contain fewer additives, preservatives, or contaminants that can interfere with nutrient absorption or metabolism. Natural or minimally processed foods can be identified by reading the ingredient list and nutrition label of the food products and choosing those that have fewer and simpler ingredients and lower amounts of sodium, sugar, and saturated fat.

- **Prepare and cook foods properly:** Preparing and cooking foods properly can enhance the bioavailability of some nutrients, as they can improve the digestibility and solubility of the nutrients and substances. Preparing and cooking foods properly can also reduce the loss or degradation of some nutrients and substances that can occur during storage, processing, or heating. Preparing and cooking foods properly can involve different methods, such as soaking, sprouting, fermenting, peeling, chopping, blending, boiling, steaming, roasting, or frying. Preparing and cooking foods properly can also involve different times, temperatures, and utensils, depending on the type and amount of the food and the desired outcome. Preparing and cooking foods properly can be learned by following the instructions and recommendations of reliable sources, such as cookbooks, websites, or experts.

- **Eat foods at the right time and frequency:** Eating foods at the right time and frequency can enhance the bioavailability of some nutrients, as they can optimize the availability and utilization of the nutrients and substances. Eating foods at the right time and frequency can also prevent the competition or interference of some nutrients and substances that can occur when they are consumed together or separately. Eating foods at the right time and frequency can involve different factors, such as the circadian rhythm, the meal pattern, the portion size, and the nutrient combination. Eating foods at the right time and frequency can be determined by listening to your body and its signals, such as hunger, satiety, energy, and mood. Eating foods at the right time and frequency can also be guided by following the recommendations and suggestions of reliable sources, such as the DGAs, the MyPlate, or the Healthy Eating Plate.

CHAPTER 8

CRAFTING A BALANCED DIET: INTEGRATING VITAMINS D, C, AND IODINE

A balanced diet is one that provides adequate amounts of all the nutrients that are essential for health and well-being. Among these nutrients are vitamins and minerals, which play important roles in various physiological processes, such as metabolism, immunity, growth, and development. Three of these micronutrients that are often lacking in the diets of many people are vitamin D, vitamin C, and iodine. In this essay, I will discuss the functions, sources, and recommendations of these three nutrients and how they can be integrated into a balanced diet. Vitamin D is a fat-soluble vitamin that is mainly involved in regulating calcium and phosphorus homeostasis and thus maintaining bone health. Vitamin D can be synthesized by the skin when exposed to sunlight or obtained from dietary sources such as oily fish, eggs, fortified foods, and supplements. The recommended daily intake of vitamin D for adults and children aged 5 years and over is 10 micrograms (µg) per day, and for infants and children under 5 years, it is 8.5 to 10 µg per day. However, due to factors such as low sun exposure, skin pigmentation, and dietary habits, many people do not meet these requirements, especially during the autumn and winter months. Therefore, it is advised to take a daily vitamin D supplement during this period and to include vitamin D-rich foods in the diet throughout the year. Vitamin C is a water-soluble vitamin that acts as an antioxidant, a cofactor for various enzymes, and a modulator of immune function. Vitamin C is found in many fruits and vegetables, such as citrus fruits, berries, peppers, broccoli, and potatoes. The recommended daily intake of vitamin C for adults is 40 milligrams (mg) per day, and for children, it is 30 to 35 mg per day. Vitamin C is easily destroyed by heat, light, and oxygen, so it is important to consume fresh, raw, or lightly cooked foods that contain vitamin C and to avoid prolonged storage or processing. Vitamin C can also be taken as a supplement, but excessive intake can cause adverse effects such as diarrhea, nausea, and kidney stones.

Therefore, it is preferable to obtain vitamin C from natural sources and to limit the supplement dose to no more than 1000 mg per day.

Iodine is a trace mineral that is essential for the synthesis of thyroid hormones, which regulate metabolism, growth, and development. Iodine is mainly found in seafood, dairy products, iodized salt, and seaweed. The recommended daily intake of iodine for adults is 150 µg per day, and for children, it is 90 to 120 µg per day. Iodine deficiency can cause goiter, cretinism, and impaired cognitive function, while iodine excess can cause thyroid dysfunction and autoimmune thyroid disease. Therefore, it is important to monitor iodine intake and status, especially for vulnerable groups such as pregnant and lactating women, infants, and people with thyroid disorders. A low-iodine diet, defined as less than 100 µg per day, has been shown to help thyroid autoimmunity, while a high-iodine diet, defined as more than 1100 µg per day, has been shown to increase the risk of thyroid disease. A moderate iodine intake, around 450 µg per day, is considered optimal for thyroid health.

Incorporating seafood into your diet

Seafood is a term that encompasses various types of fish and shellfish, such as salmon, tuna, shrimp, oysters, and mussels. Seafood is not only delicious but also nutritious, as it provides many health benefits for the body and the brain. In this section, I will explain why and how to incorporate seafood into your diet, as well as some of the best seafood choices to consume.

Why eat seafood?

Seafood is an excellent source of protein, which is essential for building and repairing muscles, organs, and tissues. Seafood is also low in saturated fat and cholesterol, which can help lower the risk of heart disease and stroke. Moreover, seafood is rich in omega-3 fatty acids, which are beneficial for the brain, the eyes, and the nervous system. Omega-3 fatty acids can improve cognitive function, memory, mood, and learning, as well as prevent or treat depression, anxiety, ADHD, and Alzheimer's disease. Omega-3 fatty acids can also reduce inflammation, which is associated with many chronic diseases such as arthritis, asthma, and diabetes.

Seafood also contains many vitamins and minerals that are vital for health and well-being. Some of these include vitamin D, vitamin B12, vitamin A, iron, iodine, selenium, and zinc. Immunity, mood management, and bone health all depend on vitamin D.Vitamin B12 is involved in the production of red blood cells, DNA, and nerve function. Vitamin A is essential for vision, skin, and mucous membranes. Immunity, mood management, and bone health all depend on vitamin D.

The transport of oxygen and the creation of energy require iron. Iodine is crucial for thyroid function and metabolism. Selenium is an antioxidant that protects the cells from damage and supports the immune system. Zinc is necessary for wound healing, growth, and immunity.

How do I eat seafood?

According to the Dietary Guidelines for Americans, it is recommended to eat at least two servings of seafood per week, or about 8 ounces for adults. One serving is equivalent to 3 ounces of cooked seafood, or about the size of a deck of cards. Children, pregnant and lactating women, and older adults may have different needs, so it is advisable to consult with a doctor or a dietitian for individual guidance.

There are many ways to incorporate seafood into your diet, such as grilling, baking, broiling, steaming, or poaching. Seafood can be eaten as a main dish, a salad, a sandwich, a soup, or a snack. Seafood can also be combined with other foods, such as vegetables, fruits, grains, nuts, seeds, herbs, and spices, to create delicious and balanced meals.

Some examples of seafood dishes are:

- Grilled salmon with roasted vegetables
- Shrimp stir-fry with brown rice

- Tuna salad with mixed greens

- Seaweed salad as a side dish

- Smoked oysters and mussels with crackers and lemon

What are the best choices for seafood?

Not all seafood is created equal, as some types may have higher or lower levels of nutrients, contaminants, or environmental impact.

Therefore, it is important to choose seafood wisely and to vary the types and sources of seafood to get the most benefits and avoid potential risks. Some of the best choices of seafood are those that are high in omega-3 fatty acids, low in mercury, and sustainably caught or farmed. Mercury is a toxic metal that can accumulate in fish and shellfish and harm the brain and nervous system, especially in fetuses, infants, and children. Some of the seafood that are high in mercury are shark, swordfish, king mackerel, and tilefish, and should be avoided or limited by pregnant and breastfeeding women and young children. Some of the seafood that are low in mercury are salmon, trout, herring, sardines, anchovies, shrimp, scallops, crab, clams, and oysters, and they can be eaten regularly by most people.

Sustainability is another factor to consider when choosing seafood, as some fishing and aquaculture practices can harm the environment, wildlife, and communities. Some of the issues include overfishing, bycatch, habitat destruction, pollution, and human rights violations.

To choose seafood that is environmentally and socially responsible, it is advisable to look for labels or certifications that indicate the seafood is wild-caught or farmed according to certain standards, such as the Marine Stewardship Council (MSC), the Aquaculture Stewardship Council (ASC), the Best Aquaculture Practices (BAP), or the Global Aquaculture Alliance (GAA). Alternatively, one can consult online guides or apps, such as Seafood Watch, FishChoice, or Seafood Selector, that provide information and recommendations on the sustainability of different types of seafood.

Seafood is a nutritious and healthy food that can provide many benefits for the body and the brain. By incorporating seafood into your diet, you can improve your protein intake, lower your risk of heart disease and stroke, enhance your cognitive function and mood, and support your immune system and overall health. However, not all seafood is equally beneficial or safe, so it is important to choose seafood that is high in omega-3 fatty acids, low in mercury, and sustainably caught or farmed. By doing so, you can enjoy the delicious and diverse flavors of seafood while protecting your health and the environment.

Building a Nutrient-Rich Plate

A nutrient-rich plate is one that provides a variety of foods that are rich in vitamins, minerals, antioxidants, and other beneficial compounds that support health and well-being. A nutrient-rich plate can help prevent or manage chronic diseases, such as diabetes, heart disease, and cancer, as well as enhance energy, mood, and performance. In this essay, I will explain how to build a nutrient-rich plate using the following steps:

- Choose a colorful and diverse array of fruits and vegetables.
- Include whole grains, legumes, nuts, and seeds as sources of complex carbohydrates and fiber.
- Select lean protein foods, such as fish, poultry, eggs, dairy, and soy products.
- Add healthy fats, such as olive oil, avocado, and nuts.
- Limit added sugars, salt, and processed foods.
- Drink water, tea, coffee, or low-fat milk.
- Choose a colorful and diverse array of fruits and vegetables.

Fruits and vegetables are the stars of a nutrient-rich plate, as they provide a plethora of phytochemicals, such as carotenoids, flavonoids, polyphenols, and glucosinolates, that have anti-inflammatory, antioxidant, and anti-cancer properties. Fruits and vegetables also provide vitamins, such as vitamin C, vitamin A, and folate, and minerals, such as potassium, magnesium, and iron, that are essential for various bodily functions. Moreover, fruits and vegetables are high in water and fiber, which can help with hydration, digestion, and satiety.

To maximize the benefits of fruits and vegetables, it is recommended to eat at least five servings per day and to choose a variety of colors, such as green, red, orange, yellow, purple, and white. Each color represents a different group of phytochemicals that have different effects on the body. For example, green vegetables, such as broccoli, kale, and spinach, contain glucosinolates that can modulate detoxification and hormone metabolism. Red fruits, such as tomatoes, watermelon, and strawberries, contain lycopene and anthocyanins that can protect against oxidative stress and inflammation.

Orange and yellow fruits and vegetables, such as carrots, pumpkin, and citrus fruits, contain carotenoids that can enhance immune function and vision.

Include whole grains, legumes, nuts, and seeds as sources of complex carbohydrates and fiber.

Whole grains, legumes, nuts, and seeds are important sources of complex carbohydrates and fiber, which can provide sustained energy, regulate blood sugar, and lower cholesterol levels. Complex carbohydrates are composed of long chains of glucose molecules that are slowly digested and absorbed by the body, unlike simple carbohydrates, such as sugar and refined flour, that are quickly broken down and cause spikes and crashes in blood sugar. Fiber is the indigestible part of plant foods that can help with bowel movements, prevent constipation, and feed the beneficial bacteria in the gut. Whole grains, such as oats, barley, quinoa, and brown rice, are grains that have not been processed to remove their bran and germ, which contain most of the nutrients and fiber. Legumes, such as beans, lentils, peas, and soybeans, are seeds that are rich in protein, iron, folate, and phytoestrogens.

Nuts, such as almonds, walnuts, pistachios, and cashews, are fruits that are high in healthy fats, protein, magnesium, and antioxidants. Seeds, such as flaxseeds, chia seeds, sunflower seeds, and pumpkin seeds, are embryonic plants that are packed with fiber, omega-3 fatty acids, and lignans.

To include more whole grains, legumes, nuts, and seeds in your diet, you can:

- Use whole-grain versions of rice, pasta, and white bread instead.
- Add beans, lentils, or soy products to soups, salads, or casseroles.
- Snack on nuts or seeds, or use them as toppings for yogurt, oatmeal, or salads.
- Sprinkle flaxseeds or chia seeds on smoothies, cereals, or baked goods.

Select lean protein foods, such as fish, poultry, eggs, dairy, and soy products.

Protein is a macronutrient that is essential for building and repairing muscles, organs, and tissues. Protein also plays a role in hormone production, enzyme activity, immune function, and fluid balance. Protein is composed of amino acids, which are the building blocks of life. There are 20 amino acids, of which nine are essential, meaning they cannot be synthesized by the body and must be obtained from food. Lean protein foods are those that have a high proportion of protein and a low proportion of fat, especially saturated fat, which can raise the risk of heart disease and stroke. Lean protein foods include fish, poultry, eggs, dairy, and soy products, which can provide complete protein, meaning they contain all nine essential amino acids. Fish, especially fatty fish, such as salmon, tuna, and sardines, are also rich in omega-3 fatty acids, which can lower inflammation and improve brain health. Poultry, such as chicken and turkey, is low in fat and high in protein, iron, and zinc. Eggs are a versatile and inexpensive source of protein, choline, and lutein. Dairy products, such as milk, yogurt, and cheese, are good sources of protein, calcium, and vitamin D. Soy products, such as tofu, tempeh, and edamame, are plant-based sources of protein, isoflavones, and fiber.

To select lean protein foods, you can:

- Choose fish or poultry over red meat, and avoid processed meats such as bacon and sausage.

- Trim the fat off the meat and remove the skin and visible fat from the poultry.

- Cook protein foods using low-fat methods, such as grilling, baking, broiling, or steaming.

- Choose low-fat or fat-free dairy products or fortified soy alternatives.

- Incorporate soy products into your meals, such as tofu stir-fry, tempeh burgers, or edamame salad.

Add healthy fats, such as olive oil, avocado, and nuts.

Fats are another macronutrient that is important for health and well-being. Fats provide energy, cushion organs, insulate the body, and facilitate the absorption of fat-soluble vitamins, such as vitamin A, D, E, and K. Fats are also the main components of cell membranes, hormones, and nerve signals. However, not all fats are created equal, as some fats can have beneficial or harmful effects on the body.

Personalized Dietary Recommendations

Diet is one of the most important factors that influence health and well-being. However, there is no one-size-fits-all diet that works for everyone, as each person has different needs, preferences, and characteristics that affect their response to food. Personalized dietary recommendations are based on the idea that nutrition can be tailored to the individual, taking into account their genetic makeup, metabolic profile, microbiome, lifestyle, and health goals. In this essay, I will explain the concept, methods, and benefits of personalized dietary recommendations and how they can help people achieve optimal health and prevent or treat chronic diseases.

What are Personalized Dietary Recommendations?

Personalized dietary recommendations are dietary advice, products, or services that are designed specifically for a person based on their unique information. Personalized dietary recommendations aim to help individuals achieve a lasting dietary behavior change that is beneficial for health. Personalized dietary recommendations are part of the broader field of personalized nutrition, which also includes personalized nutrition education, assessment, and intervention. Personalized dietary recommendations differ from general, population-based dietary guidelines, which are based on the average response of a large group of people to a certain diet or nutrient. While general dietary guidelines are useful for public health purposes, they may not be suitable or effective for everyone, as there is considerable variation in how individuals respond to food. For example, some people may have higher or lower blood glucose or triglyceride levels after eating the same meal, depending on their genetic, metabolic, and microbiome factors. Some people may also have different food preferences, allergies, intolerances, or ethical values that affect their dietary choices. Therefore, personalized dietary recommendations can provide more accurate and relevant advice that matches the individual's needs and goals.

How are Personalized Dietary Recommendations Made?

Personalized dietary recommendations are made by using various types of data and methods to assess the individual's characteristics and dietary response. Some of the data and methods that are used include:

- **Genetic testing:** Genetic testing analyzes the individual's DNA to identify variations or mutations in genes that are related to nutrition and health. For example, some genetic variants can affect the metabolism, absorption, or utilization of certain nutrients, such as folate, vitamin B12, iron, or caffeine. Some genetic variants can also influence the risk of developing certain diseases, such as obesity, diabetes, or cardiovascular disease, which may require dietary modification. Genetic testing can provide information on an individual's genetic predisposition and potential response to different dietary interventions.

- **Metabolic testing:** Metabolic testing measures the individual's biochemical markers, such as blood glucose, cholesterol, triglycerides, insulin, or inflammatory cytokines, to evaluate their metabolic status and risk of metabolic disorders. Metabolic testing can also monitor the individual's metabolic response to different foods or diets, such as the glycemic index, glycemic load, or postprandial lipemia. Metabolic testing can provide information on the individual's current health condition and metabolic flexibility and help identify the optimal macronutrient composition and portion size for their diet.

- **Microbiome testing:** Microbiome testing analyzes the individual's gut microbiota, which are the trillions of bacteria, fungi, viruses, and other microorganisms that live in the digestive tract. The gut microbiota can affect various aspects of health and disease, such as digestion, immunity, inflammation, mood, and weight. The gut microbiota can also influence the individual's response to food, as different types and amounts of bacteria can produce different metabolites from the same food, such as short-chain fatty acids, bile acids, or neurotransmitters. Microbiome testing can provide information on an individual's gut health and diversity and help determine the best foods or probiotics to modulate their microbiome.

- **Lifestyle assessment:** A lifestyle assessment evaluates the individual's lifestyle factors, such as physical activity, sleep, stress, smoking, alcohol, or medication use, that can affect their nutrition and health. Lifestyle factors can influence an individual's energy expenditure, appetite, food intake, nutrient requirements, and disease risk. Lifestyle assessment can provide information on the individual's lifestyle habits and behaviors and help identify areas that need improvement or adjustment.

- **Health goal setting:** Health goal setting involves setting specific, measurable, achievable, realistic, and time-bound (SMART) goals for the individual's health and well-being. Health goals can vary depending on the individual's needs and preferences, such as weight loss, blood pressure control, blood sugar management, or

cholesterol reduction. Health goal setting can provide motivation and direction for an individual's dietary change and help monitor their progress and outcomes. Based on the data and methods described above, personalized dietary recommendations can be generated using algorithms, models, or expert systems that integrate and analyze the individual's information and provide tailored dietary advice, products, or services. For example, some personalized dietary recommendations may suggest specific foods, nutrients, or supplements to include or avoid in the diet based on the individual's genetic, metabolic, or microbiome profile.

Benefits of Personalized Dietary Recommendations

Personalized dietary recommendations can offer several benefits for the individual and the society, such as:

- **Improved health outcomes:** Personalized dietary recommendations can help prevent or treat chronic diseases, such as obesity, diabetes, cardiovascular disease, and cancer, by providing the optimal diet for the individual's genetic, metabolic, and microbiome profile. Personalized dietary recommendations can also improve the individual's energy, mood, and performance, by providing the adequate nutrients and calories for their lifestyle and health goals.
- **Increased adherence and satisfaction:** Personalized dietary recommendations can increase the individual's adherence and satisfaction with their diet, by taking into account their food preferences, allergies, intolerances, and ethical values. Personalized dietary recommendations can also provide feedback, support, and motivation for the individual's dietary change, by monitoring their progress and outcomes, and adjusting their recommendations accordingly.

- **Reduced waste and cost:** Personalized dietary recommendations can reduce the waste and cost of food, by providing the appropriate portion size and nutrient composition for the individual's needs and goals. Personalized dietary recommendations can also reduce the waste and cost of health care, by preventing or reducing the need for medication, hospitalization, or surgery, due to improved health outcomes.

CHAPTER 9

EMPOWERING YOUR HEALTH JOURNEY: PRACTICAL TIPS AND LIFESTYLE STRATEGIES

Health is not a destination, but a journey. It is a dynamic and ongoing process that involves making choices and taking actions that support your physical, mental, and emotional well-being. However, health is not something that you can achieve overnight or by following a one-size-fits-all formula. Health is personal and unique to each individual, and it requires a holistic and proactive approach that considers your needs, preferences, goals, and challenges. In this essay, I will share some practical tips and lifestyle strategies that can help you empower your health journey and enhance your quality of life.

Define Your Health Vision and Values.

The first step to empowering your health journey is to define your health vision and values. Your health vision is a clear and compelling picture of what health means to you and what you want to achieve or experience in your health journey. Your health values are the core beliefs and principles that guide your health decisions and actions. For example, your health vision may be to have more energy, vitality, and joy in your life, and your health values may include balance, self-care, and respect.

To define your health vision and values, you can ask yourself some questions, such as:

- What are my health goals and aspirations?
- What are the benefits of achieving my health goals?
- How do I want to feel physically, mentally, and emotionally?
- What are the health behaviors and habits that support my health vision?
- What are the health barriers and challenges that hinder my health vision?
- What are the health resources and supports that facilitate my health vision?

- What are the health priorities and trade-offs that I need to consider in my health journey?

By defining your health vision and values, you can create a personal health roadmap that aligns with your purpose and passion and motivates you to take action.

Assess Your Health Status and Needs.

The second step to empowering your health journey is to assess your health status and needs. Your health status is the current condition of your health, which can be measured by various indicators, such as your body mass index, blood pressure, blood sugar, cholesterol, and other biomarkers. Your health needs are the areas of improvement or intervention that you need to address in order to achieve your health vision and values. For example, your health status may indicate that you have high blood pressure, and your health need may be to lower your sodium intake and increase your physical activity.

To assess your health status and needs, you can use various tools and methods, such as:

- **Health screenings and tests:** Health screenings and tests are procedures that can detect or diagnose health problems, such as diabetes, hypertension, or cancer. Health screenings and tests can help you identify your health risks and take preventive or corrective measures. You can consult with your doctor or health care provider to determine the appropriate health screenings and tests for you based on your age, gender, family history, and other factors.
- **Health questionnaires and surveys:** Health questionnaires and surveys are instruments that can measure your health behaviors, attitudes, and perceptions, such as your dietary intake, physical activity, stress level, or satisfaction with your health. Health questionnaires and surveys can help you evaluate your health strengths and weaknesses and identify your health opportunities and threats. You can find various health questionnaires and surveys online or create your own based on your health vision and values.

- **Health trackers and apps:** Health trackers and apps are devices or applications that can monitor and record your health data, such as your steps, calories, sleep, or heart rate. Health trackers and apps can help you track your health progress and performance and provide feedback and guidance. You can choose from a variety of health trackers and apps, depending on your health goals and preferences.

By assessing your health status and needs, you can establish a baseline and a benchmark for your health journey and set realistic and specific health goals.

Implementing Sustainable Lifestyle Changes

Sustainable lifestyle changes are changes in the way we live, work, and consume that aim to reduce our environmental impact and enhance our well-being. Sustainable lifestyle changes can help us address the global challenges of climate change, biodiversity loss, and pollution, as well as improve our health, happiness, and quality of life. However, implementing sustainable lifestyle changes can be difficult, as they may require breaking old habits, overcoming barriers, and adapting to new situations. In this essay, I will provide some practical tips and strategies that can help us implement sustainable lifestyle changes in our daily lives.

Identify Your Motivation and Goals.

The first step to implementing sustainable lifestyle changes is to identify your motivation and goals. Your motivation is the reason why you want to make sustainable lifestyle changes, such as protecting the environment, saving money, or improving your health. Your goals are the specific and measurable outcomes that you want to achieve by making sustainable lifestyle changes, such as reducing your carbon footprint, saving a certain amount of money, or lowering your blood pressure. By identifying your motivation and goals, you can clarify your purpose and direction and increase your commitment and motivation.

To identify your motivation and goals, you can ask yourself some questions, such as:

- What are the benefits of making sustainable lifestyle changes for myself, others, and the planet?
- What are the costs or risks of not making sustainable lifestyle changes for myself, others, and the planet?
- What are the sustainable lifestyle changes that I want to make, and why?
- How will I measure and monitor my progress and achievements?

Start Small and Build Up.

The second step to implementing sustainable lifestyle changes is to start small and build up. Starting small means making simple and easy changes that can have a significant impact, such as switching to LED light bulbs, using reusable bags, or taking shorter showers. Building up means gradually increasing the frequency, intensity, and duration of your sustainable lifestyle changes, such as walking or cycling more often, buying more organic or local food, or volunteering for environmental causes. By starting small and building up, you can avoid overwhelm and frustration and build confidence and momentum.

To start small and build up, you can use some strategies, such as:

- Break down your goals into smaller and more manageable steps, and prioritize them according to their importance and urgency.
- Set a realistic and flexible timeline for your sustainable lifestyle changes, and adjust it as needed.
- Celebrate your achievements and reward yourself for your efforts, such as by treating yourself to a movie, a massage, or a new book.
- Learn from your mistakes and challenges, and use them as opportunities to improve and grow.

Seek Support and Collaboration.

The third step to implementing sustainable lifestyle changes is to seek support and collaboration. Seeking support means reaching out to others who can help you with your sustainable lifestyle changes, such as your family, friends, co-workers, or experts. Seeking collaboration means joining or creating groups or communities that share your vision and values, such as online forums, local clubs, or social movements. By seeking support and collaboration, you can gain information, inspiration, and encouragement and overcome isolation and resistance.

To seek support and collaboration, you can use some methods, such as:

- Communicate your motivation and goals to others and ask for their feedback, advice, or assistance.
- Invite others to join you in your sustainable lifestyle changes, and make them fun and enjoyable, such as by having a potluck, a swap party, or a game night.
- Participate in events or activities that promote sustainable lifestyles, such as workshops, webinars, campaigns, or rallies.
- Share your experiences and stories with others, and learn from their experiences and stories.

Long-Term Wellness and Nutrient Maintenance

Wellness is a state of optimal physical, mental, and emotional well-being that enables one to live a fulfilling and meaningful life. Nutrient maintenance is the process of ensuring adequate intake and utilization of essential nutrients that support the body's functions and health. Long-term wellness and nutrient maintenance are interrelated and interdependent, as nutrition is a key factor that influences wellness, and wellness is a key factor that influences nutrition. In this essay, I will discuss the importance, challenges, and strategies of long-term wellness and nutrient maintenance and how they can enhance one's quality of life.

The Importance of Long-Term Wellness and Nutrient Maintenance

Long-term wellness and nutrient maintenance are important for various reasons, such as:

- **Preventing or managing chronic diseases:** Many chronic diseases, such as obesity, diabetes, cardiovascular disease, and cancer, are largely influenced by nutrition and lifestyle factors.

- By maintaining a balanced and varied diet that provides adequate amounts of macronutrients (carbohydrates, proteins, and fats) and micronutrients (vitamins and minerals), one can reduce the risk or severity of these diseases. Moreover, by adopting healthy lifestyle habits, such as regular physical activity, stress management, and adequate sleep, one can enhance the body's ability to use and regulate nutrients and improve the body's immune system and resilience.

- **Promoting growth and development:** Nutrition and wellness are especially important for growth and development during the life stages of infancy, childhood, adolescence, pregnancy, and lactation. During these periods, the body has increased nutrient requirements and demands, and any deficiency or excess can have lasting consequences on the body's structure and function. For example, inadequate intake of iron, iodine, or folate can impair cognitive development and learning, while excessive intake of sugar, salt, or fat can increase the risk of obesity and metabolic disorders.

- **Supporting aging and longevity:** Nutrition and wellness are also important for aging and longevity, as they can help prevent or delay the onset of age-related diseases and disabilities, such as osteoporosis, arthritis, dementia, and frailty. By consuming foods that are rich in antioxidants, anti-inflammatory, and anti-aging compounds, such as fruits, vegetables, nuts, seeds, and fish, one can protect the cells and tissues from oxidative stress and inflammation and enhance the body's repair and regeneration mechanisms. Furthermore, by engaging in physical, mental, and social activities, one can maintain the body's strength, flexibility, and coordination and preserve the brain's function and memory.

Challenges of Long-Term Wellness and Nutrient Maintenance

Long-term wellness and nutrient maintenance are not easy to achieve, as they face various challenges, such as:

- **Environmental factors:** The environment can affect one's nutrition and wellness in many ways, such as by influencing the availability, accessibility, affordability, and quality of food, water, and air. For example, climate change, pollution, and natural disasters can reduce the production and diversity of crops, increase the contamination and scarcity of water, and worsen the air quality and temperature. These factors can compromise one's nutrition and wellness and increase exposure to toxins and pathogens.

- **Social factors:** society can affect one's nutrition and wellness in many ways, such as by influencing the norms, values, beliefs, and behaviors of individuals and groups. For example, culture, religion, education, media, and peer pressure can shape one's food preferences, choices, and practices and affect one's nutritional status and health outcomes. These factors can also create social inequalities and disparities in nutrition and wellness and affect one's access to resources and opportunities.

- **Personal factors:** The individual can affect one's nutrition and wellness in many ways, such as by influencing the knowledge, skills, attitudes, and motivations of oneself and others. For example, genetics, metabolism, microbiome, and health conditions can affect one's nutrient needs and responses and require personalized and tailored nutrition and wellness interventions. Moreover, emotions, habits, and preferences can affect one's dietary and lifestyle patterns and pose barriers or facilitators to nutrition and wellness change.

Strategies For Long-Term Wellness and Nutrient Maintenance

Long-term wellness and nutrient maintenance are possible to achieve, as they can be supported by various strategies, such as:

- **Evidence-based guidelines:** Evidence-based guidelines are recommendations that are based on scientific research and expert consensus and provide general and specific guidance on nutrition and wellness for different populations and situations. For example, the Dietary Guidelines for Americans[1] and the Physical Activity Guidelines for Americans are evidence-based guidelines that provide advice on what and how much to eat and drink and how and how much to move for optimal health and well-being. By following evidence-based guidelines, one can obtain reliable and relevant information and direction on nutrition and wellness.

- **Personalized interventions:** Personalized interventions are actions that are based on individual data and feedback and provide customized and adaptive nutrition and wellness solutions for different needs and goals. For example, genetic testing, metabolic testing, microbiome testing, and lifestyle assessment are methods that can provide individual data on one's nutrient requirements and responses and help design personalized interventions, such as dietary supplements, food products, or services. By using personalized interventions, one can obtain accurate and effective nutrition and wellness outcomes.

- **Supportive environments:** supportive environments are settings that are based on collective actions and policies and provide conducive and sustainable nutrition and wellness opportunities for different contexts and communities. For example, schools, workplaces, health care facilities, and public spaces are settings that can provide collective actions and policies, such as nutrition education, food labeling, menu planning, food safety, physical activity promotion, and environmental protection. By creating supportive environments, one can obtain accessible and affordable nutrition and wellness resources and support.

Conclusion

In this book, we have explored the benefits of ample vitamin C, vitamin D, and iodine for our health and well-being. We have learned how these three nutrients interact and synergize with each other and how they affect various aspects of our body's functions and health, such as bone health, immune function, thyroid function, cognitive performance, and aging. We have also learned how to optimize our nutrient intake and uptake by understanding the factors that influence nutrient synthesis, absorption, and utilization, such as sunlight exposure, food combinations, bioavailability, and genetic, metabolic, and microbiome variations. Moreover, we have learned how to craft a balanced diet that integrates vitamins C, D, and iodine and how to personalize our dietary recommendations based on our individual needs and goals. Finally, we have learned how to empower our health journey by implementing sustainable lifestyle changes, such as physical activity, stress management, and sleep hygiene, and how to maintain our wellness and nutrient status in the long term.

We hope that this book has provided you with valuable information and practical tips on how to maximize your health and well-being by exploring the benefits of ample vitamin D, vitamin C, and iodine. We also hope that this book has inspired you to take action and make positive changes in your diet and lifestyle that can enhance your quality of life. Remember, health is not a destination, but a journey. It is a dynamic and ongoing process that involves making choices and taking actions that support your physical, mental, and emotional well-being. By reading this book, you have taken the first step in your health journey. The next step is up to you. We encourage you to apply what you have learned from this book and to continue learning and experimenting with your nutrition and wellness. We wish you all the best in your health journey, and we hope that you will share your experiences and stories with us and others. Thank you for reading this book, and we hope that you have enjoyed it as much as we have enjoyed writing it.

www.ingramcontent.com/pod-product-compliance
Lightning Source LLC
Chambersburg PA
CBHW080730260726
48660CB00010B/3781